INTRODUCTION

History of cannabis

Cannabis has a six thousand years' history that dates back to the early and middle Bronze Age.

In 4,000 BC, cannabis was a major food crop and was remarked as one of the five grains in China. In 2,737 BC, cannabis was used as a medicinal drug. This is the earliest record of it being used for medicinal purpose. Emperor Shen- Nung acknowledged its uses for treatments of over one hundred ailments. These ailments included gout, malaria, and rheumatism.

Between 2,000 and 1,400 BC, cannabis was used in steam baths by the nomadic Indo-European people. They also used it in burial rituals where cannabis seeds were burned.

In Hindu religious texts, cannabis was chronicled as a "bringer of freedom" and "source of happiness." They used it in their regular services and rituals. As its uses kept on increasing, the pathway for further research of its medicinal uses opened up during the 2,000–1,000 BC.

There is information regarding the use of cannabis as a treatment for inflammation in Egyptian medical papyrus of medical knowledge. The Assyrians noted the psychedelic effects of the use of cannabis in 900 BC.

During 450–200 BC, it is stated that there was widespread use of cannabis in the Greek Empire. It was used as a treatment for earaches and toothaches by the physician Dioscorides. In the Roman Empire, the women who were going into labor took it to alleviate the pain.

A mixture of wine and cannabis was used to anesthetize patients for the first time during AD 207. It was stated to be a beneficial treatment for epilepsy. This was researched by Arabic scholars al–Badri and al–Mayusi in AD 1,000.

Avicenna was a Persian medical writer. He published Avicenna's *The Canon of Medicine* in AD 1025. In it, he stated that cannabis could be used as a treatment for edema, headaches, gout, and infected wounds. His work influenced a lot of Western medicine after being extensively studied from the thirteenth to the nineteenth century.

In AD 1300, the Arab traders brought cannabis from India to Eastern Africa, where it was used for the treatment of many ailments. Those included dysentery, malaria, fever, and asthma. In AD 1500, the cannabis was brought to America by the Spanish. It was utilized as a source for making practical equipment, like clothes and ropes. Many years later, it was also used for its medicinal and psychotropic properties.

Napoleon introduced cannabis to France. He brought it to his homeland from Egypt in AD

1798. It was mainly used to treat cough, jaundice, and tumors. It was also analyzed for its sedative and pain-relieving qualities.

The year 1839 is marked as the year when Western medicine was introduced to the therapeutic benefits of cannabis by an Irish doctor William O'Shaughnessy. He came to the conclusion that cannabis bears no negative effects. After that, medicinal usage and research on cannabis rose exponentially.

Medicinal cannabis was used in 1900 for the treatment of ailments like rheumatism, labor pain, and nausea. It was available as "Piso's cure" and "one- day cough cure." In 1914, the Harrison Narcotics Tax Act was passed. It established drug use to be a crime in the United States. In 1937, the Marijuana Tax Act was passed; it declared that all sales and use of cannabis were banned in the United States. In 1964, an Israeli chemist discovered and synthesized the THC. THC is an active component of cannabis.

In 1970, the plant cannabis was listed as "having no accepted medicinal use." In the United States, cannabis was categorized as a schedule 1 drug. This limited any further research into the plant. In 1988, cannabinoid receptors CBD1 and CBD2 were discovered. They are the most significant number of neuro receptors present in the brain.

During the years 2000 to 2018, many governments were allowing the use of cannabis for its medicinal purposes. It is only legalized for use when obtained from a legalized producer. Its use for recreational purposes is becoming common, and its legalization is imminent in many countries.

The medicinal use of cannabis has a long and rich history. Due to regulations and restrictions on the use of cannabis, the research on it has been severely affected. We are way more behind than we should be on the research regarding cannabis. Many studies and proofs are required to clarify the status of cannabis as a favorable product once and for all.

In October of 2017, a report was published by the World Health Organization. It was a preview report that compiled all the current and potential purposes or uses of CBD. CBD is now supported to be used in the treatment of Dravet syndrome. There are still more pieces of evidence that can appear as the research on this topic expands.

According to the WHO, cannabis could potentially open new gates to the treatment of extremely fatal diseases like Parkinson's, Alzheimer's, and Huntington's. Cancer, depression, multiple sclerosis, psychosis, and anxiety treatments stand to gain from CBD. You can learn more details on CBD with different diseases later in this book.

CBD

Cannabidiol (CBD) is present among the hundred compounds that are found in the cannabis plant. These compounds are known as phytocannabinoids. CBD is produced in tiny hairs that stick out from the cannabis plant's flowers and leaves. It is also stored in those parts that are known as trichomes. Trichomes are attached to flowers and leaves of the cannabis plant.

The endocannabinoid system is responsible for maintaining many psychological processes in the human body. The cannabinoids interact with it and influence it. Some of the methods it affects are pain, inflammation, learning, and emotions. Between CBD and THC, the latter can cause a sort of high. It affects the behavior of cells of the brain and body. It also changes the communication between these two types of cells.

CBD has a mellowing effect and doesn't cause a high. It is proclaimed to have anti-inflammatory and pain-reduction effects. At this stage, there are only a few studies done on pure CBD that can be extracted from the cannabis plant. It can be consumed in an oil or pill form.

Researchers are still trying to figure out the exact quantity of CBD and THC to utilize for various medicinal purposes. The studies about figuring dosage and their effects are still ongoing.

Uses of CBD

Many researchers in this day and age are seeking alternatives to regular pharmaceuticals. They want a respite from the side effects of regular medicine that is administered today, a medication that is provided by nature so that it doesn't pose harm to our body.

Some researchers and doctors claim there are not enough studies to support the claims of CBD's medicinal purposes. They are still not completely aware of their effects on the human mind and body. They say that CBD can trigger many different things in different receptors. Most, however, acknowledge that CBD does have anti-inflammatory and pain reducing properties.

The potential for its medicinal uses and benefits is immense and unprecedented. It can single-handedly change the medicine world forever

- People use it in oil form to treat common minor afflictions like a sore joint or a rash.

- Some users also use it to alleviate anxiety. It helps them feel calm.

- It is also claimed to treat many different ailments. These include eczema, joint pain, acne, and insomnia.

- The neuroprotective effects of CBD are proven (Hampson, Grimaldi, Axelrod, and Wink,

1998).[1]

- The anti-cancer properties that make people very interested and curious about it are still under research ("Studies on CBD and Cancer," 2019).[2]

[1] Hampson, A.; Grimaldi, M.; Axelrod, J.; and Wink, D. (1998). "Cannabidiol and (-) 9-tetrahydrocannabinol Are Neuroprotective Antioxidants." *Proceedings of the National Academy of Sciences*, 95(14), 8268-8273. DOI: 10.1073/pnas.95.14.8268.

[2] "Studies on CBD and Cancer" (2019). Retrieved from https://www.projectcbd.org/cancer.

THC

THC is mainly a compound present in a cannabis plant that comes from Marijuana. Its abbreviation is tetrahydrocannabinol. It is responsible for the high that is caused by consuming marijuana. THC is one of the cannabinoids and most widely known as well. Cannabinoids interact with the brain and the body's receptors.

An Israeli chemist, Raphael Mechoulam, was the one to isolate THC in 1964. He isolated THC from Lebanese hashish. It was then the research on cannabis really took off. Many other cannabinoids were also discovered after that along with endocannabinoids and cannabinoid receptors that are present throughout the whole body. Endocannabinoids are compounds that are similar to THC. They are naturally made by our body to maintain its health and stability.

Cannabinoid receptors are present in abundance in some areas of the brain. These areas of the brain are linked to thinking, pleasure, memory, time perception, and coordination. THC combines with these receptors and causes them to activate. When this happens, then a person's thinking, memory, coordination, and sensory as well as time perception are all affected ("Marijuana," 2019).[3]

THC is structure-wise similar to natural chemical anandamide. It is produced by the brain. THC is found in the resin that is secreted by lands of a Marijuana cannabis plant. THC activates and stimulates cells present in the brain. It causes them to release dopamine, which can cause euphoria ("How Does Marijuana Produce Its Effects?" 2019).[4]

Hippocampus is the area of the brain that produces new memories. It affects the information processing part in the hippocampus region. THC can cause delusions and hallucinations. A person begins to experience them after thirty minutes of consumption. Its effects last about two hours. After the consequences of being high have worn off, the psychomotor impairment may still persist.

Uses of THC

THC is also linked with some side effects. Those are elation, short-term memory loss, sedation, tachycardia, and anxiety. There are also some users who claim the pain-relieving effects of the THC. There are many medicinal and recreational uses of THC.

- There are many ways to consume THC. It can be used internally in syrups, edibles, and oils or externally with the application of lotions and balms for its anti-inflammatory properties.

---

[3] "Marijuana" (2019). Retrieved from
https://www.drugabuse.gov/drugs-abuse/marijuana.

[4] "How Does Marijuana Produce Its Effects?" (2019). Retrieved from
https://www.drugabuse.gov/publications/research-reports/marijuana/how-does-marijuana-produce-its-effects.

- It can also reduce anxiety and has pain-relieving effects on dogs.

There is only one FDA-approved medicine that is produced from synthetic THC called Marinol.

The Difference in THC and CBD

These two compounds have very similar chemical structure. They are both parts of the cannabis plant and are extracted from it. THC causes one to feel high. CBD balances out the potent effects of THC. CBD is associated with an increase in energy while THC can cause ecstasy. CBD tones down the effects caused by THC.

CBD versus THC Medical Uses

Medical Uses of CBD	Medical Uses of THC
Anti-seizure	Analgesic
Analgesic	Anti-nausea effects
Anti-tumor properties	Aid in sleeping
Antipsychotic	Anti-anxiety
Anti-inflammatory	Muscle spasticity
Depression	

Difference between CBD Oil and Hemp Oil

Hemp oil and CBD oil vary hugely by their uses.

CBD oil is a cannabidiol-enriched cannabis oil. The hemp oil, meanwhile, is made from its seeds. They both come from the same plant. They both have ingredients that are being investigated for their medicinal purposes. They are both used for different reasons. Most people confuse them both and believe they are both the same thing.

Hemp-derived CBD oil is produced from stalks, leaves, and flowers of the hemp. Mostly, the strains are picked for extracting CBD oil as they contain higher CBD levels. Making CBD oil from strains also increases the potency of the product. CBD products that come from natural and organic whole plant cannabis (Hemp) are recommended mostly. It is safer than the ones made from industrial hemp.

In recent years, the popularity of CBD oil (Hemp) has risen exponentially. Its use for medicinal purposes is highly sought after now more than ever before. It is beneficial for many ailments. It doesn't have the intoxicating effect of Marijuana, but it has all its medicinal advantages. It is used for the treatment of many neurodegenerative and inflammatory disorders. It is also beneficial for epilepsy treatment.

Hemp oil is taken from seeds of the hemp plant. Industrial hemp is the only one utilized for producing hemp oil. Its psychedelic effects are reduced to a minimal. One of the uses of hemp oil includes cooking as it is packed with nutrients. It can also be used as an olive-oil replacement in salads.

Hemp oil can also be used as a moisturizer for its specific properties. It can also act as a base form for a variety of plastic. It is used as an alternative for petroleum. It can also be used as a biodiesel fuel just as any other vegetable oil. Hemp oils are also used in the production of different soaps and lotions. Some foods also contain hemp oil...

Projection of CBD Business

If the cannabis industry keeps on growing at its current rate, then by 2020, the American market will reach $20 billion. The Brightfield Group, a cannabis industry analyst, has claimed that the Hemp-CBD industry alone is expanding at an extraordinary rate and could reach $22 billion by 2022 ("CBD Worth $22 Billion by 2022? That's Crazy, Right?" 2019).[5]

This is as recent as 2017–2018, the CBD

products have hit the local markets and stores. They are coming in the form of many different types of products. The numbers that the industry hit in 2018 was projected to be around $500 million. That number could go up to forty times in the next four years. The CBD market doubled in size over the past couple of years, and the trend doesn't seem likely to stop.

CBD industry is experiencing such growth because it doesn't have the challenges of traditional cannabis. The legalization and logistic issues of traditional cannabis hinder its industry growth significantly.

There are also a lot of studies and research currently going into the CBD. Substantial investment is being brought in the field of CBD research to find ways to grasp different markets. CVS and Walgreens are two major retailers that are going to cover topical CBD products. This industry has suddenly bloomed on the scene out of nowhere. The CBD market has been expanding majorly on a mouth-to-mouth basis.

2018 Farm Bill and Its Impact on the Hemp Industry

Marijuana is a schedule 1 narcotic as stated by the FDA. Hemp and cannabis are mainly cousins. Hemp is a low THC and high CBD content. The 2018 farm bill has legalized on a federal level the commercial production of hemp.

On December 20, 2018, the president passed the farm bill. The Hemp Farming Act of 2018 was also included in this bill. This bill legalizes hemp production and usage all across the nation. The legal state, however, is not altered due to this bill. Many businesses are gearing up to make a profit by utilizing the possibilities of CBD.

That is why investors are funding into researchers because they also want to profit from it as well. This may create an influx of CBD products all over the nation. The CBD-infused stuff is very likely to have prices that are not standardized. These products will not go through a system of check and balance, so we are likely not getting factual information regarding the quality and quantity of CBD in a product.

The 2018 farm bill amends the term *marijuana* to exclude hemp. This term was founded in 1972 Controlled Substances Act. Hemp was defined as the cannabis plant, which has less than 0.3 percent of THC. Below are some of the potential uses of hemp, other than CBD products

Below are some of the potential uses of hemp, other than CBD products

- A sweater that is more durable than cotton and softer than any fabric you have come across.

- A car with lighter-than-a-steel structure. It can stand almost ten times the amount of impact of steel, and it would not even dent.

- A single acre of the fast-growing plant can replace the paper that is produced from four acres of trees.

America has suppressed many potential jobs and research that could transform essential products. They can make products that are more environmentally sustainable.

---

[5] "CBD Worth $22 Billion by 2022? That's Crazy, Right?" (2019). Retrieved from https://www.brightfieldgro up.com/post/cbd-worth-22-billion-by-2022.

THE SCIENCE BEHIND CBD

Humans have utilized the cannabis plant since ancient times. It has been used throughout history and all over the world from Asia to Europe. Cannabis is a genus that consists of three psychoactive plants:

- Cannabis sativa

- Cannabis indica

- Cannabis ruderalis

People claim a lot of health benefits of cannabis. Its advantages include treatments for a range of ailments, from nausea to immune system problems. One might ask these questions: "If cannabis is so highly regarded for its health-related advantages, then why isn't there more particular studies and proof of them? Why is there not enough scientific evidence to deny or back these claims?" The main reason behind the lack of knowledge on this subject is that in 1970, America scheduled it as a schedule 1 drug. This meant that it was included in the same category as heroin, ecstasy, and LSD. They are all highly addictive substances that are illegal in most countries. They were classified as having "no accepted medical use," and it was also stated that they pose a risk and high potential for abuse. This categorization made cannabis unsuitable for research in the laboratory. There was a risk involved in committing a federal offense.

In some states, cannabis has been given the green light for medicinal and recreational use. The pro- and anti-cannabis communities are at odds with each other, and this has become the topic of many debates. One side wants it banned permanently while the other party wants it to be accessible everywhere. CBD, or cannabidiol, is sort of like a hot topic since it has come on the scene with an unprecedented potential for a revolution of many industries.

It single-handedly makes a lot of industries efficient and sustainable. Its uses are still being researched.

Tetrahydrocannabinol (THC)   Cannabidiol (CBD)

The structural formulas of Tetrahydrocannabinol (THC) and Cannabidiol (CBD).

The structural formula of THC and CBD ("CBD vs. THC: What Are the Main Differences?" 2019)[6]

CBD was first isolated in 1940. There is a family of over 113 bicyclic and tricyclic cannabinoid compounds that are naturally found in the cannabis. CBD is one of those compounds. Its molecular formula ($C_{21}H_{30}O_2$)

is similar to THC. This formula represents that both CBD and THC have twenty-one carbons, thirty hydrogens, and two atoms of oxygen. The molecular mass is also very similar as THC has a mass of 314.469 g/mol, and CBD has a mass of 314.464 g/mol.

The cannabigerolic acid (CBGA) is a forerunner for all the cannabinoids that occur naturally. The CBDA synthase cyclizes CBGA into cannabidiolic acid. This acid form then undergoes decarboxylation to bring out the final product of CBD. CBD contains a hydroxyl group while THC contains a cyclic ring. CBD has low solubility in water. However, it is readily soluble in organic solvents, lipids, and alcohol.

CB1 is a G protein-paired cannabinoid receptor. It is present in the central and peripheral nervous system. It occurs in ample quantity in the brain. CB1 is a part of the endocannabinoid system, and endogenous neurotransmitters are responsible for its activation. These neurotransmitters are anandamide and 2- arachidonoylglycerol along with a few other naturally occurring compounds. Phytocannabinoids, which are present in cannabis, are also neurotransmitters. THC stimulates the CB1 receptors as it is a potent partial agonist of CB1. This leads to one experiencing the psychoactive effects when one tends to consume cannabis.

CBD is labeled as a negative allosteric modulator of CB1 (Laprairie, Bagher, Kelly, and Denovan-Wright, 2015).[7]

---

[6] "CBD vs. THC: What Are the Main Differences?" (2019). Retrieved from https://www.analyticalcannabis.com/articles/cbd-vs-thc-what-are-the-main-differences-297486.

[7] Laprairie, R.; Bagher, A.; Kelly, M.; and Denovan-Wright, E. (2015). "Cannabidiol Is a Negative Allosteric Modulator of the Cannabinoid CB1 Receptor." *British Journal of Pharmacology*, 172(20), 4790–4805. DOI: 10.1111/bph.1325

It is an established fact that CBD is a non-intoxicating compound. In recent years, CBD has sparked a lot of interest among physicians and scientists. There is still ongoing research on CBD's effects on a molecular level that makes it so beneficial to human and pet's health.

Cannabidiol is a pleiotropic drug. It produces various effects through multiple molecular pathways present in our body. The scientific literature till now has discovered over sixty-five molecular targets of the CBD. CBD binds to a minimal extent with CB1 and CB2, two cannabinoid receptors. CBD does inflect many non-cannabinoid receptors and the ion channels. CBD also acts via many pathways that don't require any receptor. An example of this is that it delays the restoration of anandamide and adenosine, which are endogenous neurotransmitters.

CBD binds to the nuclear receptors present in the human body, and it is a plant compound so one might wonder, how does this all come about?

CBD, first of all, has to go through the cell membrane. It does so by traveling with the FABP, which is an abbreviation of fatty-acid-binding proteins. These intracellular transport molecules are also responsible for transporting THC and endocannabinoids to various targets within the cells.

Here are some of how CBD imparts its various remedial effects on the human body.

1. Serotonin Receptors

In the University of São Paulo and King College, the researchers have carried out a study related to CBD and how it can have a positive effect on anxiety. This was pioneering research on the subject (Schier et al., 2014). CBD activates the 5-HT1A (hydroxytryptamine) serotonin receptor. This gives us an indication of CBD's anti-anxiety effects.

The 5-HT1A belongs to the family of 5-HT receptors. They are present in the central and peripheral nervous system. These receptors are only activated by the neurotransmitter serotonin. The 5-HT receptors are behind the torrent of chemical messages. It triggers the signals that produce responses that could either be excitatory or inhibitory.

CBDA stands for cannabidiolic acid. It is the raw and unheated type of CBD that occurs in the cannabis plant. CBDA has a stronger affinity toward 5-HT1A receptor than CBD. CBDA is an effective antiemetic. It is believed to be more potent than CBD and THC, which are also effective against nausea.

2. GPR55-Orphan Receptors

As CBD activates some receptors and ion channels. There are also new studies that suggest that CBD also acts as a hindrance because it can also block and deactivate G protein-coupled receptors, which are known as GPR55.

GRP55 is also referred to as an orphan receptor because scientists are not sure about its origin. They don't know whether it belongs to some other family of receptors. GPR55 is present in the cerebellum and throughout the brain in abundance. It regulates physiological processes, like bone density and blood pressure.

GPR55 stimulates the osteoclast cell function. This function aids bone reabsorption. When the GPR55 receptor is overactive, then this may be an indicator of osteoporosis.

GPR55 is also revealed in many different types of cancers. When GPR55 has activated, it boosts the proliferation of cancer cells (Hu et al., 2019).[8]

CBD acts as the enemy of GPR55. Both of the processes—bone reabsorption and cancer cell proliferation—are subsided by halting the GPR55 receptor

signaling (Whyte et al., 2009).[9]

3. PPARS-Nuclear Receptors

CBD activates the PPARs that are present on the surface of the cell's nucleus. PPARs are an abbreviation of *peroxisome proliferator-activated receptors*. By enabling the PPARs, CBD depicts its anti-cancer properties.

Anti-proliferative effects are observed when the PPAR-gamma receptor is activated. Its activation also regresses the tumor in human lung cancer cells. PPAR-gamma activation decreases the amyloid-beta plaque. It is known as the key molecule related to Alzheimer's development.

---

[8] Hu, G.; Ren, G.; Shi, Y.; A, A.; PF, S.; and RJ, R. et al. (2019). "The Putative Cannabinoid Receptor GPR55 Promotes Cancer Cell Proliferation." Retrieved from https://www.nature.com/articles/onc2010502.

[9] Whyte, L.; Ryberg, E.; Sims, N.; Ridge, S.; Mackie, K.; and Greasley, P. et al. (2009). "The Putative Cannabinoid Receptor GPR55 Affects Osteoclast Function in Vitro and Bone Mass in Vivo." *Proceedings of the National Academy of Sciences*, 106(38), 16511-16516. DOI: 10.1073/pnas.0902743106.

This is how CBD is known to be beneficial to the sufferers of Alzheimer's disease. The main reason for it is that CBD is a PPAR-gamma agonist.

PPAR receptors are also involved in the modulation of specific genes. The genes are involved in lipid uptake, energy homeostasis, insulin sensitivity, and other metabolic activities.

4. Vanilloid Receptors

CBD brings on therapeutic properties, which it carries out through numerous ion channels. TRPV1 receptors bind with CBD, and they operate as an ion channel. TRPV1 receptors are known to moderate conditions like inflammation, body temperature, and pain perception.

TRPV is an abbreviation of *transient receptor potential cation channel subfamily V*. There many dozens of TRP subfamilies, and TRPV1 is also one of them. They are responsible for bringing in the effects of many medicinal herbs. Scientists call TRPV1 as vanilloid receptors. The name comes from a vanilla bean. CBD binds to TRPV1, which has an impact on pain perception. Anandamide is also a TRPV1 agonist.

5. The Reuptake Inhibitor

Cannabidiol can make a strong connection with three types of FABPs. CBD opposes the endocannabinoids for the same transport molecules. Once they get inside the cells, anandamide is broken down by fatty acid amide hydrolase, or FAAH, as a part of the molecular life cycle. The FAAH is a metabolic enzyme. The CBD, however, hinders this process by decreasing the anandamide access to FABP transport molecules. This also causes a delay of endocannabinoid transfer inside the interior of the cell.

CBD acts as anandamide reuptake and breakdown inhibitor (Deutsch, 2016).[10]

This causes the endocannabinoid levels in the brain's synapses to rise. CBD's function as a reuptake inhibitor increases the endocannabinoid tone. This is the main reason why CBD is lauded for its neuroprotective effects, especially seizures.

CBD also inhibits the adenosine reuptake. It has anti-inflammatory and anti- anxiety effects that are linked to this mechanism. CBD boosts the adenosine levels in the brain by deterring the reuptake of adenosine. This regulated the adenosine receptor activity in the brain. A1A and A2A adenosine receptors play an essential role in cardiovascular function. They act to control myocardial oxygen consumption and blood flow.

---

[10] Deutsch, D. (2016). "A Personal Retrospective: Elevating Anandamide (AEA) by Targeting Fatty Acid Amide Hydrolase (FAAH) and the Fatty Acid Binding Proteins (FABPs)." *Frontiers in Pharmacology*, 7. DOI: 10.3389/fphar.2016.00370.

6. Allosteric modulator

Cannabidiol also acts as an allosteric receptor modulator. It means that it is capable of changing the shape of the receptor. By doing so, it can affect the signal transmission of the receptor by either enhancing it or inhibiting it.

Scientists in Australia suggest that the CBD functions as a "positive allosteric modulator" of the GABA-A receptor (Bakas et al., 2017).[11]

This means that the CBD influences GABA-A in such a way that amplifies the receptor-binding affinity. Mainly, the association for its principal endogenous agonist, gamma-aminobutyric acid (GABA), is boosted. GABA is known as the primary inhibitory neurotransmitter of the central nervous system. The interceding of the sedating effects of Benzos is carried out by GABA receptor transmission. CBD acts as anti-anxiety because it alters the shape of the GABA-A receptor in a certain way. This alteration of forms boosts the natural calming effect of GABA.

CBD has also been identified to function as a "negative allosteric modulator" of the cannabinoid CB1 receptor. This receptor is present in large amounts in the central nervous system and the brain. CBD doesn't bind readily to the CB1 receptor. It interacts allosterically with it and changes its shape. This causes the ability of CB1 to bind with THC to weaken it. By doing this, it mitigates the THC's psychotropic ability. That is why it doesn't cause a high when people use CBD-enriched cannabis as compared to THC-dominant drug. So that is why CBD-rich products can impart several health benefits without causing any dysphoric effect.

---

[11] Bakas, T.; van Nieuwenhuijzen, P.; Devenish, S.; McGregor, I.; Arnold, J.; and Chebib, M. (2017). "The Direct Actions of Cannabidiol and 2-arachidonoyl Gglycerol at GABA-A Receptors." Pharmacological Research, 119, 358- 370. DOI: 10.1016/j.phrs.2017.02.022

Terms Related to Cannabis

One thing that you might find difficult in keeping up with is the terminology. Many words are similar but have a very different meaning. There are some main terms listed here that will help just in case.

Cannabinoids: They belong to a diversified chemical family. They also have a lot of variety of uses. Some are considered illegal while others have soothing and relaxing properties.

CBD: CBD is a cannabinoid that occurs naturally. It comes in second as the most abundant component of the cannabis plant. It is legal and safe to consume, unlike THC.

THC: It is the compound that is found in the most amount in the marijuana cannabis plant. It is a potent psychotropic cannabinoid. Its production and usage are under strict regulation because it causes a high after consumption of marijuana.

Cannabis: Cannabis is a flowering plant. It is used widely for its medicinal and recreational purposes. Marijuana and Hemp are both part of the Cannabis family.

Marijuana: The Marijuana plant has broad leaves, and has more like a bushy, short appearance.

Hemp: The Hemp plant has skinny and tall leaves, and most of the leaves are on the top of the plant.

CBD Oil from Marijuana: Contains about 10 % CBD and 20 % THC

CBD Oil from Hemp: Contains about 20 % CBD and less than 0.3 % THC

Can You Fail a Drug Test after Consumption of CBD?

The THC amount in CBD from Hemp is less than 0.3 percent. It will not show on tests to be positive for THC. However, if you consume about 1,000–2,000 mg per day of

CBD, then you can fail a drug test for THC. This is according to SAMHSA guidelines. SAMHSA is the abbreviation of Substance Abuse and Mental Health Services Administration.

If you use a hemp-derived product and consume high doses of CBD, then there is a low risk of failing the THC test if you are tested regularly. An alternative to using hemp-derived products is purified CBD. Purified or isolate CBD only contains CBD and no other compounds. There are more advantages to using CBD oil than purified CBD.

Even from taking high doses of CBD oil, one cannot get high. Our coordination, balance, and motor functions are not at risk of compromise from using CBD oil. The psychedelic effects start to appear when the 3–5 percent amount of THC is consumed. CBD only has 0.3 percent amount of THC. There is no case or report of hallucinations caused by using CBD oil. It augments the sense of well-being and does not leave us distraught.

CBD Extraction Methods and Which One Is the Best?

Cannabinoids are extracted from hemp. They are then typically concentrated into an oil form. When we consume this, it can make cannabinoids amounts to increase for a continuous period in our blood levels. This effect makes CBD much healthier to use for recreational purposes as compared to vaporized marijuana. This is because the latter one diffuses from the blood very quickly as compared to the former.

There are four ways to extract the CBD.

CO_2 extraction method:

This is a relatively newer method that does not utilize any chemicals, so instead of chemical solvents, it uses carbon dioxide. This method involves extracting the chemical components from the flower buds. The next step that follows is the distillation, where they blend into a thick oil.

Chemical extraction method:

This is the most generic method for CBD extraction. In this method, we utilize solvents that typically are hexane or alcohol. The dense oil and some harmful residue are left behind after the solvent dries off.

Lipid-based extraction:

In this method, we use fats that absorb the chemical compounds of cannabis. After incorporating them, they also enclose the compounds within itself. Organic coconut oil is one of the fats you can use in this method. The main advantage of this method is that the presence of fats makes the product easier to consume. This bioavailability makes this process much safer than extraction from chemicals.

Vapor or thermal distillation:

In this distillation method, hot air is employed to obtain chemical compounds from the plant. Hot air vaporizes the chemical compounds from the buds. These vapors are then distilled into CBD oil. Cannabinoids are also activated by using this method. The extra carboxyl ring is removed from the molecular chain, which helps it to interact with CB receptors promptly. This ensures ultimate medicinal usage of the CBD and the method that enables it is known as decarboxylation.

It is the best method to obtain all the range of chemical compounds found in the cannabis plant. Another advantage of this method is that we get terpenes, which are also very beneficial. Terpenes can cause an entourage effect, which helps enhance the effects of CBD more than other methods.

THE USES OF CBD

CBD for Anxiety and Stress

Around two thousand years ago, the use of cannabis and CBD for anxiety first made an appearance in a Vedic text. This particular use of the plant is prevalent across many cultures. THC can elevate the feeling of anxiety in some patients and decrease it in others. CBD has a much more consistent effect on anxiety as compared to THC. CBD has shown over and over again a reduction in anxiety. The stress-related effects of the CBD are linked to the activity in some regions of the brain, especially the limbic and paralimbic areas. A 2012 research has concluded that CBD cause reduction of anxiety (Stress, 2019).[12]

A review was published in *Neurotherapeutics* found out that CBD can be beneficial for people who suffer from anxiety. CBD was found out to be useful in some disorders that are linked to anxiety. Since CBD can cause a reduction of anxiety, it is also possible that these disorders that are heavily related to anxiety could also benefit from CBD. Some of these include panic disorder, general anxiety disorder, social anxiety disorder, post-traumatic stress disorder (PTSD), and obsessive-compulsive disorder (Blessing, Steenkamp, Manzanares and Marmar, 2015).[13]

---

[12] Stress, P. (2019). "The 10 Most Powerful Essential Oils on the Planet for Relieving Anxiety & Stress.: Retrieved from https://www.consciouslifestylemag.com/best-essential-oils-for-anxiety-and-stress/.

[13] Blessing, E.; Steenkamp, M.; Manzanares, J.; & Marmar, C. (2015). "Cannabidiol as a Potential Treatment for Anxiety Disorders." *Neurotherapeutics*, 12(4), 825-836. DOI: 10.1007/s13311-015-0387-1.

The current treatments for these disorders have a considerable number of side effects that cause more problems than they can overcome. Since then, multiple studies have been carried out to get closer to having more evidence to cement this property of CBD. Some animal-related studies revealed that if the endocannabinoid system is boosted, it can alleviate the consequences of stress, both behavioral and physical.

High-CBD cannabinoids can have positive effects in lessening temporary stress and also chronic anxiety. It provides protection for the body against the harsh physiological effects of stress and anxiety.

There is a lot of confusion on how to get and what is the proper dosage and delivery methods when taking cannabidiol. You can consult a medical practitioner who is experienced with medicinal cannabis. CBD products with a ratio of 20:1 or higher are suggested for anxiety. The methods you can use to consume the CBD are drops, edibles, or capsules. All these methods have their own pros and cons, so choose the way that suits you the best.

You should always start with a micro dose and move up slowly. Make sure not to go above the recommended dosage range. When you feel that your symptoms are diminishing, this means that the dosage is working for you. If you want immediate relief from an anxiety or panic attack, put drops directly under your tongue, smoking or vaporizing also work well. These are methods through which CBD gives a very direct effect.

The cannabis health index (CHI) is a scoring system for cannabis in general. It is based on evidence and effectiveness on numerous health problems. It is based on the research data that is currently available, so based on this CHI, the treatment of anxiety by CBD is in a *possible to the probable range*.

CBD for Depression and Mood Disorders

Clinical depression is a severe type of mood disorder. It is accompanied by sadness, decreased appetite, loss of interest in things, and a decrease in energy. In some cases, it brings about suicidal thoughts in a person.

Serotonin is a chemical messenger that is believed to function as a mood stabilizer. It is commonly used in the medicines that are administered for depression. The endocannabinoid system's neural network is similar in the function to dopamine and serotonin. Cannabinoids, like THC, also affect the serotonin levels. A small dose of THC increases serotonin while a high dosage can cause the serotonin levels to drop. Some studies have also suggested that CBD should be represented as a possible antidepressant drug. It can enhance serotonergic and glutamate signaling

("Cannabis: Potent Anti-depressant in Low Doses, Worsens Depression at High Doses," 2019).[14]

According to the cannabis health index (CHI), the cannabis treatment for depression is *rated in the range of "possible to probable."* Studies until now have indicated positive effects and potential for effective treatment of depression by using CBD.

Studies on animals have indicated that the CBD acted as an anti-anxiety and anti-depressant in multiple models. The CBD compound worked by combining with the 5-HT1A neuro-receptor. CBD works to improve the functionality of the endocannabinoid system. It increases the time in which anandamide works on the CB1 and CB2 receptors.

---

[14] "Cannabis: Potent Anti-depressant in Low Doses, Worsens Depression at High Doses" (2019). Retrieved from https://www.sciencedaily.com/releases/2007/10/071023183937.html.

The primary role of the anandamide is to maintain the balance through inhibiting or enhancement when the levels increase or decrease respectively. The levels of substances it controls include dopamine, serotonin, GABA-glutamate systems, etc. This is one of the main reasons that CBD is linked to modulate depression and stress.

CBD for Brain Health

Cannabinoids are also known as the neuro-protectors. They aid in regulating the health of the brain. They are linked to multiple functions and the effects that they can have on the brain. Some tasks that the cannabinoids perform are the removal of damaged cells and the increase in the productivity of the mitochondria.

The presence of extra glutamate stimulates the nerve cells present in the brains. It causes the cells to become hyper - and overstimulated. This can lead to cell damage. CBD works to mitigate the toxicity caused by glutamate. Cannabinoids protect the brain cells against damage (Brain, 2019).[15] Some studies have also stated that CBD can have an anti-inflammatory effect on the brain, but the evidence is inconclusive.

With age, the brain grows old as well. The process of development of new neurons slow down. New cells are needed to regulate mental health. They are also essential to prevent degenerative diseases from occurring. A study conducted in 2008 showed that the small number of cannabinoids, like CBD and THC, boosted the development of new nerve cells in the animals. This phenomenon was observed not only in young brains but also in the older ones.

---

[15] Brain, T. (2019). "The Keys to Brain Health: 10 Supplements and Habits That Supercharge Your Brain." Retrieved from https://www.consciouslifestylemag.com/brain-health-key-supplements-habits/.

CBD and Pain

In 1859, Sir John Russell Reynolds stated that there is no better option than cannabis for relieving certain types of pain. He was a physician to the queen and a well-known epilepsy research pioneer. Cannabis has been used in almost all the cultures from across Europe to Asia, specifically to relieve pain. For many different kinds of pain, cannabis is an effective remedy and a safe analgesic. The research on this topic is also ongoing.

CBD use for pain is the most common among the masses. The general perception is that it is a more natural alternative to pain medications. Scientists differentiate the pain into two types. One is neuropathic, which is a chronic type of pain. Another is nociceptive pain, which usually happens for only a limited amount of time. Cannabis seems to affect both of these types of pain. The endocannabinoid system is shown to be involved in the processing of the pain signals as some studies have shown us. Finding the right dosage is very important if you want to experience any benefits from the CBD.

CBD for Inflammation

A lot of studies have indicated that CBD has anti-inflammatory properties. It can help reduce inflammation as it interacts with the endocannabinoid system present in organs throughout the human body. Inflammation is involved in a lot of diseases.

A study was conducted on mice and rats, and the researchers found out that CBD reduced the chronic pain and inflammation in them (Xiong et al., 2012).[16]

---

[16] Xiong, W.; Cui, T.; Cheng, K.; Yang, F.; Chen, S.; Willenbring, D.; et al. (2012). "Cannabinoids Suppress Inflammatory and Neuropathic Pain by Targeting α3 Glycine Receptors." *The Journal of Experimental Medicine*, 209(6), 1121–1134. DOI: 10.1084/jem.20120242.

The anti-inflammatory properties of the CBD make it able to help in so many other health-related conditions. It is believed that CBD's anti-inflammatory effects are related to its ability to interact with specific receptors present in the immune cells. CB2 receptors are present inside the immune cells. The CBD promptly interacts with it. CBD can stimulate these receptors. Upon activation, a large variety of immune responses are triggered. One of those immune responses is to fight off inflammation present in the body.

CBD for Skin Health

CB2 receptors are present in high concentration in the skin. CBD oil is also being manufactured in the form of lotions, serum, or salve. The antioxidant in the CBD oil has many advantages. It can repair the damage that is caused by the harmful UV rays on the skin. The topical products that are based on cannabis are being evolved to treat other skin problems as well. They are developed to have an effect on ailments like acne, psoriasis and other skin problems. It can also boost the process of healing of the damaged skin.

History of cannabis indicates that it was commonly utilized for the treatment of wounds in both animals and humans. The new research nowadays is finding new ways to combat acne with CBD. Medical science has advanced so far, yet there is no standard medication for acne that eradicates it forever. CBD is well known for its various properties that are proving beneficial as new research and evidence emerge. Some claim that CBD may prove to be more effective than vitamin C or E. Both of these vitamins are essential for good skin health. Today, there are many topical products that promise to treat and prevent skin cancers.

Topical application of the CBD and THC has been linked to treatment of some certain skin cancers, such as melanoma and carcinoma. The use of CBD oils for treating skin inflictions is gaining rapid popularity. Rick Simpson claims to have cured his basal cell carcinoma by using cannabis oil. He now has a whole line of products related to CBD. The cannabis is not psychoactive when we apply it topically.

CBD for Bone Health

Cannabinoids are known to aid in the bone metabolism process. Bone metabolism is a cycle of our body in which the old bone material is replaced by the new one at a rate of about 10 percent per year. This process is significant in maintaining healthy and strong bones.

CBD has been shown to inhibit an enzyme that is responsible for ruining the bone-building elements in the body. This way, CBD also helps with diseases of bones, like osteoporosis and osteoarthritis, which are related to age. In these diseases, the body no longer produces the new bone and cartilage cells.

CBD is linked with triggering the process of new bone formation. It has also been found to speed up the process of healing the broken bones. Due to the creation of a stronger fracture callus, the likelihood of breaking the bone again is significantly reduced.

CBD for Cancer

Cancer is a deadly disease. After so many advancements and research on this disease, we still haven't found an effective treatment that doesn't include its harsh side effects. Even if you complete the treatment, there is a risk involved that cancer could come back again.

When the word got around that CBD could potentially be effective against cancer, people were immediately interested in it. The reason being that the current treatments of cancer are often a nightmare. A study done in 2012 showed that the animals that were given CBD are less likely to develop colon cancers. They were introduced to carcinogens in a laboratory after undergoing treatment by CBD.

There are many studies that show that THC can be helpful with preventing and reduction of tumors. In 2015, 84,000 medical records were investigated by scientists. They all belonged to male patients based in California. The scientists found out that those who used cannabis had a bladder cancer rate that was 45 percent below the normal.

There is still a lot of research that is being carried out on this topic. If we find concrete proof and evidence that cannabis is indeed the solution to cancer, it could change the medical world forever. Cancer won't be a death sentence to a person anymore. Cannabis could revolutionize the treatment of this nightmare. The research that is being carried out is mostly focusing on the ratio of CBD to THC. Researchers are figuring out the best quantity of both substances to utilize in the medication for different types of cancer. Dose level for cancer prevention and treatment is also under heavy research.

CBD and Cardiovascular Disease

There are a couple of studies that depict the effectiveness of cannabis for regulating cholesterol. In 2013, 4,652 people participated in a study about the effect of cannabis on cardiovascular health. They compared the metabolic systems of non-users, current users, and former users. The current users were found out to have elevated blood levels of high-density lipoprotein (HDL-C), which is also known as the good cholesterol.

In the same year, another study was carried out in Canada. They analyzed over seven hundred members of Canada's Inuit community. They concluded that regular cannabis users have higher levels of the HDL-C and reduced levels of LDL-C. LDL-C is bad cholesterol.

Atherosclerosis is a disease that commonly occurs in Western nation typically due to their lifestyle and diet regime. It can cause a stroke or lead to heart disease. Atherosclerosis is a chronic inflammatory disorder. This disease includes depositing of the atherosclerotic plaques. Atherosclerotic plaques are the immune cells that carry oxidized LDL. There are some shreds of evidence found that suggest that endocannabinoid signals play an essential role in the pathology of atherogenesis.

The condition is caused as a response to the injuries in the arterial walls' lining. These injuries are caused by high blood pressure, infectious microbes, or a high amount of homocysteine, which is an amino acid. There are some existing treatments for these conditions, but they are not without the harmful side effects.

An animal trial was carried out in 2005 that showed that a low dose of cannabinoids reduced the progression of atherosclerosis. Next year, the scientists suggested that the immunomodulatory capacity of the cannabinoids is established in the world of science. They also said that the cannabinoids have a vast potential for a variety of conditions of the human body.

Another animal study was carried out in 2007. This study also showed that CBD has a positive effect on cardiac-related problems. It was found out even to have a cardioprotective impact during a heart attack.

cannabinoids reduced the progression of atherosclerosis. Next year, the scientists suggested that the immunomodulatory capacity of the cannabinoids is established in the world of science. They also said that the cannabinoids have a vast potential for a variety of conditions of the human body.

Another animal study was carried out in 2007. This study also showed that CBD has a positive effect on cardiac-related problems. It was found out even to have a cardioprotective impact during a heart attack.

A review was published in the British Journal of Clinical Pharmacology, stating that CBD can aid a lot in the prevention of spreading of cancer. The CBD has low levels of toxicity. It doesn't cause harm to humans. The CBD compounds were also found to deter the growth of tumor cells. They CBD can destroy the tumor cells in some cases as well (Yamini Ranchod, 2019) [17.]

CBD for Diabetes

There are several studies out there that indicate that those who use cannabis regularly have a lower body mass index, reduced risk of developing diabetes, and smaller waist circumference. A report was published in 2011 that did a survey on approximately 52,000 participants.

---

[17] Yamini Ranchod, M. (2019). "Cancer: Overview, Causes, Treatments, and Types." Retrieved from https://www.medicalnewstoday.com/articles/323648.php

The conclusion that they got from this particular study was that in cannabis users, the rates of obesity are about one-third lower than the others. This is all despite the fact that those specific participants eat more calories per day. This consumption of food could potentially be related to THC's stimulation of hormone that can increase appetite known as ghrelin. Ghrelin not only increases appetite but also boosts metabolism as well.

In 2006, a study on lab rats indicated that the use of just CBD only lowered the occurrence of diabetes in them. The research on this effect of CBD has shown us that CBD is beneficial for weight loss. They help convert the white fat into weight-reducing brown fat.

Researchers have also found out that participants of the study that were current cannabis users have insulin levels that were 16 percent lower than other participants who didn't use cannabis. These cannabis users also had 17 percent lower levels of resistance of insulin and elevated levels of HDL cholesterol that protects us against developing diabetes. This protective effect of cannabis fades with time as people stop using cannabis or don't use it as often. Those who were once cannabis users depicted similar associations that were not that noticeable.

Weight gain and obesity are brought on by excessive insulin. The higher amount of insulin boosts the conversion of sugars into stored fats. There is ongoing research about the link of CBD with obesity and type 2 diabetes. It has the potential of some major breakthrough. The study is mainly focused on the interchange between cannabinoids and regulation of insulin.

Type 1 diabetes, an auto-immune disease, could be caused by inflammation. This occurs when the cells in the pancreas are attacked by the immune system.

Research in 2016 indicated that CBD might help lower the inflammation of the pancreas (Lehmann et al., 2017).[18]

CBD for Pets

Pets, especially dogs, stand to gain a lot of positive benefits from CBD. The effects of CBD are found to be the same in humans, dogs, cats, and other pets. The reason behind this is that pets also have an endocannabinoid system that operates in the same way as the one that humans have. Many ailments that affect humans have a similar effect and symptoms on pets as well.

It is also well-known as an anti-convulsant, that is one of the most beneficial uses of CBD. It acts as a stress reliever.

---

[18] Lehmann, C.; Fisher, N.; Tugwell, B.; Szczesniak, A.; Kelly, M.; and Zhou, J. (2017). "Experimental Cannabidiol Treatment Reduces Early Pancreatic Inflammation in Type 1 Diabetes." *Clinical Hemorheology and Microcirculation*, 64(4), 655–662. DOI: 10.3233/ch-168021.

Not only does CBD help with physical conditions, but also it is beneficial for certain mental health conditions. Just like humans, pets also suffer from stress and anxiety. Although the source may be different, the symptoms are generally the same.

It also acts as a painkiller and boosts the homeostasis. CBD is very well known for its pain-killing properties. It also helps to manage pain in a variety of ways. It stops or hinders the absorption of anandamide. This leads to having lower pain sensations in the presence of more anandamide.

Some CBD benefits for dogs are listed below.

- Allergies

- Anti-inflammatory

- Anxiety

- Appetite

- Arthritis

- Fatty Tumors

- Chronic Pain

- Quality of Life

- Digestive issues

- Seizures

- Glaucoma

- Joint Issues

- Phobias

- Skin Issues

- Skin Problems

CBD for PTSD

PTSD is post-traumatic stress disorder. It can occur after a person goes through an especially severe patch in their lives. There is psychotherapy as well as medications for the treatment of PTSD.

CBD can potentially provide an excellent alternative to the medications for PTSD. These medications have serious side effects. CBD, on the other hand, has no reported or known harmful side effects. ("Post-Traumatic Stress Disorder (PTSD): Cannabinoids and CBD Research Overview," ECHO Connection, 2019).[19]

CBD improves the endocannabinoid system's regulation of vital functions. These functions include memory retrieval and consolidation. CBD is capable of activating CB1 and CB2 receptors. It can prompt the production of more neurotransmitters that are linked with improving the feeling of pleasure, happiness, and memory.

---

[19] Retrieved from https://echoconnection.org/post-traumatic-stress-disorder-ptsd-medical-cannabis-and-cbd- research-overview/.

CBD has become very popular among PTSD patients. CBD can prevent the underlying trauma from showing up. It can also effectively hinder nightmares and the traumatic memories that can be detrimental to one's emotional well- being.

CBD for Insomnia

The research that is done up till now suggests the CBD oil can help us sleep better. It can improve our sleep and can make an effective remedy for insomnia. The research on this topic is ongoing.

The leading cause of insomnia is stress. The stress levels in the population of today are at an all-time high. When we are in a prolonged state of stress, it can bring about some dangerous health conditions. These conditions may include cancer, depression, and anxiety. CBD interacts with the receptors that are present in the brain, and it improves the cognitive ability of the brain. This helps the brain massively, and the CBD can empower it to respond to stressful situations more effectively (Pava, Makriyannis, and Lovinger, 2016).[20]

CBD for Epilepsy

CBD can help reduce the symptoms of epilepsy. It can mitigate the frequency and strength of the seizures. CBD also helps in controlling spasms, tics, and tremors. We got the first proof of CBD having anticonvulsant properties.

The story came out of a girl named Charlotte. She was a young girl who suffered from an extreme case of epilepsy. Charlotte's only hope was a tincture. It ended up helping her in managing three hundred weekly seizures.

---

[20] Pava, M.; Makriyannis, A.; and Lovinger, D. (2016). "Endocannabinoid Signaling Regulates Sleep Stability." *PLOS ONE*, 11(3), e0152473. DOI: 10.1371/journal.pone.0152473.

The tincture was formed with CBD-enriched cannabis (Saundra Young, 2019).[21]

CBD for Combating Drug Addiction

CBD is a non-psychedelic compound obtained from cannabis. One of the most underrated uses of CBD is helping with the eradication of drug or alcohol addiction.

It is a bizarre approach but one that works better than other methods. There is a lot of research to back up this fact as well. If you factor in how the CBD interacts with our body's endocannabinoid system, then things start to clear up.

One week of administering CBD can prevent relapses for many months. Research has shown that with just seven days of CBD

---

[21] Saundra Young, C. (2019). "Marijuana Stops Child's Severe Seizures." CNN. Retrieved from https://edition.cnn.com/2013/08/07/health/charlotte-child-medical-marijuana/index.html.

CBD for Combating Drug Addiction

CBD is a non-psychedelic compound obtained from cannabis. One of the most underrated uses of CBD is helping with the eradication of drug or alcohol addiction.

It is a bizarre approach but one that works better than other methods. There is a lot of research to back up this fact as well. If you factor in how the CBD interacts with our body's endocannabinoid system, then things start to clear up.

One week of administering CBD can prevent relapses for many months. Research has shown that with just seven days of CBD treatment, many positive results were found. There was no development of addict-like characteristics.

It also stops the subject from relapsing for about five months (Gonzalez- Cuevas et al., 2018).[22]

a lot of research to back up this fact as well. If you factor in how the CBD interacts with our body's endocannabinoid system, then things start to clear up.

One week of administering CBD can prevent relapses for many months. Research has shown that with just seven days of CBD treatment, many positive results were found. There was no development of addict-like characteristics. It also stops the subject from relapsing for about five months (Gonzalez-Cuevas et al., 2018).[22]

[22] Gonzalez-Cuevas, G.; Martin-Fardon, R.; Kerr, T.; Stouffer, D.; Parsons, L.; Hammell, D. et al. (2018). "Unique Treatment Potential of Cannabidiol for the Prevention of Relapse to Drug Use: Preclinical Proof of Principle." *Neuropsychopharmacology*, 43(10), 2036-2045. DOI: 10.1038/s41386-018-0050-8

CHOOSE THE BEST CBD OIL AND DOSE PROPERLY

<u>Quality of CBD Oil</u>

CBD is a rapidly growing industry. The recent boom in consumption means that many companies are trying to make as much profit from selling CBD as they can. There is a high probability that not all of them are concerned with putting the best and healthiest product on the market. The CBD oil is growing in popularity, and many companies are putting different unstandardized products out there. The consumers are left confused about the reliability of the product. Here are some of the ways you can identify quality CBD oil. Also, check out what companies received the seal of approval by the U.S. Hemp Authority.

1. Ingredients

A good quality CBD oil does not have more than two or three ingredients in it. CBD doesn't work well if it is consumed purely on its own. It looks like table salt when it is in 100 percent pure form freshly extracted from the plant. It needs to be infused with oil to work effectively. By mixing up with oil, the human body can absorb it and metabolize readily. The pure CBD is absorbed lesser than the one infused with a carrier oil. A high-quality carrier oil is the most crucial ingredient to any oral cannabidiol. A good quality product will have 250–1,000 mg per fluid ounce of CBD. CBD quantity in a product may vary, so be sure to look out for the amount of CBD in the product before purchasing it. Hemp seed oil, olive oil, MCT oil and coconut oil all make up good carrier oil. However, since hemp seed oil comes from the same plant as the CBD comes from, it is probably the one that works the best.

2. Manufacturing

Different CBD brands have different extraction methods. Some methods that companies employ may be cheap ones, and they can leave behind traces of toxic solvents.

The CO_2 extraction method is expensive and more complex than the other ones. This method produces CBD oil that has retained its purity throughout the extraction process.

Some companies also utilize organic, pharmaceutical grade ethanol to extract CBD. The use of ethanol removes the toxins and residues that are left behind from the hemp plant. This extraction method has the highest yield of cannabinoids as compared to other processes. It is also considered to be one of the safest means of extraction.

So, before you go and purchase any CBD oil, do a little research on their production method. You can find this information on their website. The ones that are produced from CO_2 or ethanol methods are recommended.

3. The Source of CBD

The hemp plant is known to be a hyper-accumulator. This means it absorbs anything and everything that exists in the soil. If the ground in which hemp grew is fertile, the plant will be of good quality. Good-quality plant means good- quality CBD oil.

If the ground in which hemp plant was produced is contaminated with heavy metals, then the CBD oil produced from it will have the same heavy metals in them as well. This makes it unsafe for humans to consume.

CBD oil has a risk of developing a bad reputation because some manufacturers don't care about the quality of hemp that they use. The result is that the product they produce might be laden with toxic heavy metals.

Try to use products made from US-grown hemp. The farmers are certified by the state department of agriculture, so it is suggested that if you want to know the quality of CBD oil, research where they source their hemp from. This information should be available on the website of the retailer or the manufacturer.

4. Amount of THC in the CBD oil.

THC is responsible for the psychotropic effects caused by the intake of marijuana or agricultural hemp. Hemp is used over marijuana for the production of CBD oil because it contains lower levels of THC. The amount of THC present in hemp is meager, but it is still there and can cause psychedelic effects if it is not processed effectively. CBD oil is manufactured from hundreds of thousands of hemp-plants. If the processing of the plant is done poorly, the produced CBD oil may have a lot more amount of THC than the recommended level.

It is suggested that the amount of THC in CBD oil should not be more than 0.3 percent. You can check for this information on the label of the product.

5. Isolates or full spectrum

Good CBD oil is manufactured from using the whole plant. This ensures that the oil contains CBD and all the primary and secondary components of the hemp plant. These other components are flavonoids, terpenes, and other cannabinoids. They raise the effectivity of CBD more than if it is used just on its own.

CBD isolates contain only the Cannabidiol compound. Isolates have zero THC in them, which is great for children, or people who are getting tested for their jobs, and don't want to risk trace amounts of THC showing up in their results.

You can check the labels on the product. It

will tell you if the manufacturer used the whole plant or full spectrum.

6. Third-party test results

The brand that produces high-quality CBD always provides third-party results for their customers. The tests from independent labs will ensure the quality of the CBD oil that you are purchasing. These tests will satisfy the consumers about product reliability and whether all the claims they made are true or not. Basic things to look for are low THC, high quantity of CBD, and lack of toxins and impurities.

A good and reputable brand will always make the recent lab results available for the customers. They may be on the website or in the packaging of the product. If you cannot find the test results, make sure to contact them for it. Excellent customer service is always a sign of a good product.

The accredited laboratories to ISO/IEC

17025:2017 test CBD to make sure that it is free from the following:

- Residual harmful solvents
- Fungus or bacteria
- Pesticides
- Heavy metals
- Any other foreign material

The Dosage of CBD Oil

Use the log section in the back of this book to correctly find the best dosage for YOUR needs. Always start very low. For example, if you use a 500 mg oil, I would start with 3 – 5 drops, 2 times a day. Take notes on how you feel. Then slowly increase the dosage, until you feel better. If you start to feel worse, after an increase, lower the dosage again.

If you start with too much CBD, in rare cases it could cause Flu like symptoms, comparable to the Keto Flu, when you start out with Keto.

That's why **LESS IS MORE** AND **SLOWER is BETTER**!

The average dose of CBD can be somewhere in between 10 mg and 50 mg taken at one to three times per day. Higher doses may be used to control pain. They are tolerated by our body very well. Different products have different concentration of CBD. That is one of the reasons that some will notice effects on the lower-dose range while others may require taking more to see the same effects.

- If you take the CBD oil in liquid form, one dropper of low concentration product will give you about 3 mg CBD. This quantity is not enough to let you experience any noticeable effects. A low-concentration product is about 100 mg CBD per fluid ounce.

- A medium-concentration product has about 500 mg of CBD per fluid ounce. A medium-grade product will provide about 15 mg of CBD. This quantity of CBD is considered a good dose.

- High-concentration produce has about 1,500 mg per fluid ounce. One full dropper of this product will give you about 50 mg of CBD.

How Do You Take CBD Oils?

- **In food**

Adding CBD oil to your food makes it easier to take in. You can make your own edibles or purchase premade foods that are infused with CBD. If you make the meal yourself, then you have to take care of the amount of CBD oil to put in your food and how much you eat. Edibles take two to four hours to take effect.

Some pros of this method are that out of all other consumption methods, it has the most long-lasting effect. You have different options to choose from on how you want to consume the CBD. You can try out new shakes, food recipes, etc.

Some cons are that it can take a long time to

kick in, up to four hours. You also have to take care to ascertain the correct dose. This is especially true if you buy food or drinks that claim to have CBD in it. Usually, you just don't know.

- **Vaping**

You can also vape CBD oil with a vaporizer pen. Vaping is an alternative to smoking. It imparts the maximum possible effect without being detrimental to your throat or lungs. All though we don't know the long-term effects on vaping yet.

Some pros of this method are that it ensures optimal effect due to high concentration. You can easily monitor the amount of dose you take.

Some cons of this method are that high concentration may not be what you are looking for. It also requires you to purchase some accessories (e.g., a vape pen).

- **Capsules**

CBD can be ingested via capsules or in powder form. It passes through the digestive tract and then gets absorbed in the bloodstream. Then by blood, it can travel throughout your entire body.

Some pros of this method: This is the best way if you are looking for long- term supplementation. It can also help you control the dose of CBD oil. A con associated with this method: It takes the slowest time for CBD to reach its targets.

- **Sublingually**

CBD oil tinctures are also available, and they come in bottles that look like eye drops. You can put a few drops under your tongue and hold them in there for approximately thirty seconds. Some advantages of this method are that it is discreet and easy to use. Controlling your dosage is easy.

This method works the fastest, so if you need an immediate way to get rid of stress or pain, then you should take the CBD oil under your tongue. The effects will likely last a few hours.

Find Your Proper Dosage Level!

Many people don't know how to get the proper dosage when taking CBD Oil. Often, they take too much, so it won't help them. Everyone's body reacts differently, that's why you need to keep track of your intake, to figure out what YOUR sweet-spot is. **The key is to start low and slow!** Keep on one level for about a week, before increasing the dose by 2 – 3 drops. Check out the section about dosage in this book for more information on it.

Some people see results really fast. Other's take a little longer, so be patient.

How to Use This CBD Log Book

1. Every person in your household should use their own sheet. Write down your **name**.
2. Put in the **brand** - not all brands are created equal. You want to know if one brand helps you more or less
3. The **strength** of the CBD, for example 500 mg is a very common one. You'll find this info on the bottle.
4. **Date/Time** for when you take the drops, ideally is in the morning and at night
5. **Dose:** How many drops did you take?
6. **Peace:** Put in a checkmark if you feel at peace, no anxiety or panic attacks
7. **Sleep:** Did you fall asleep quickly, and did you have a restful night? If so, put a checkmark in there.
8. **Pain:** Did your pain-level improve? Or if you only have occasional headaches, when was the last time you had it? If you feel that it got better, please put a checkmark there.
9. **Mood:** Did your mood get better? Do you feel more balanced? Not freaking out so fast, or getting upset over little things? If so, please put a checkmark there.
10. **Skin:** Does your skin look better, less red? Did a wound heal faster? Your psoriasis not so prominent anymore? If so, please put a checkmark there.

11. Document in **Symptoms Relieved**, what symptoms have disappeared or got better, so when you look back, you'll remember everything.
12. In **Notes** write down for example if you were very stressed out for some reason, or if you were sick, on vacation etc. It is important to get the full picture.

If you need more log pages, please go to www.caromollet.com/dosage

Find Your Perfect Dosage!

Name: _____

CBD Brand: _____

CBD Strength: _____

Date/ Time	Drops	Peace	Sleep	Pain	Mood	Skin

Symptoms Relieved

Notes

Find Your Perfect Dosage!

Name:

CBD Brand:

CBD Strength:

Date/Time	Drops	Peace	Sleep	Pain	Mood	Skin

Symptoms Relieved

Notes

Find Your Perfect Dosage!

Name: _____

CBD Brand: _____

CBD Strength: _____

Date/ Time	Drops	Peace	Sleep	Pain	Mood	Skin

Symptoms Relieved   **Notes**

Find Your Perfect Dosage!

Name:

CBD Brand:

CBD Strength:

Date/Time	Drops	Peace	Sleep	Pain	Mood	Skin

Symptoms Relieved

Notes

Find Your Perfect Dosage!

Name: _____

CBD Brand: _____

CBD Strength: _____

Date/Time	Drops	Peace	Sleep	Pain	Mood	Skin

Symptoms Relieved

Notes

Find Your Perfect Dosage!

Name:

CBD Brand:

CBD Strength:

Date/Time	Drops	Peace	Sleep	Pain	Mood	Skin

Symptoms Relieved

Notes

Find Your Perfect Dosage!

Name:

CBD Brand:

CBD Strength:

Date/ Time	Drops	Peace	Sleep	Pain	Mood	Skin

Symptoms Relieved

Notes

Find Your Perfect Dosage!

Name: _____

CBD Brand: _____

CBD Strength: _____

Date/ Time	Drops	Peace	Sleep	Pain	Mood	Skin

Symptoms Relieved

Notes

Find Your Perfect Dosage!

Name: _____

CBD Brand: _____

CBD Strength: _____

Date/ Time	Drops	Peace	Sleep	Pain	Mood	Skin

Symptoms Relieved

Notes

Find Your Perfect Dosage!

Name:

CBD Brand:

CBD Strength:

Date/Time	Drops	Peace	Sleep	Pain	Mood	Skin

Symptoms Relieved

Notes

Find Your Perfect Dosage!

Name:

CBD Brand:

CBD Strength:

Date/ Time	Drops	Peace	Sleep	Pain	Mood	Skin

Symptoms Relieved   **Notes**

Find Your Perfect Dosage!

Name: _____

CBD Brand: _____

CBD Strength: _____

Date/Time	Drops	Peace	Sleep	Pain	Mood	Skin

Symptoms Relieved

Notes

Find Your Perfect Dosage!

Name:

CBD Brand:

CBD Strength:

Date/ Time	Drops	Peace	Sleep	Pain	Mood	Skin

Symptoms Relieved

Notes

Find Your Perfect Dosage!

Name: _____

CBD Brand: _____

CBD Strength: _____

Date/Time	Drops	Peace	Sleep	Pain	Mood	Skin

Symptoms Relieved

Notes